ANTI PARKII
DISEASES DIET
COOKBOOK

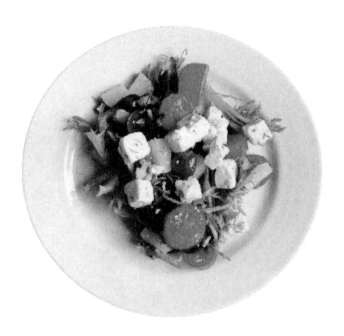

DR. PENNY WATSON

Copyright © 2023 by Dr. Penny Watson

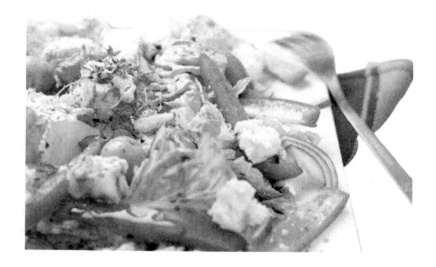

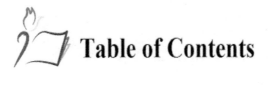

Table of Contents

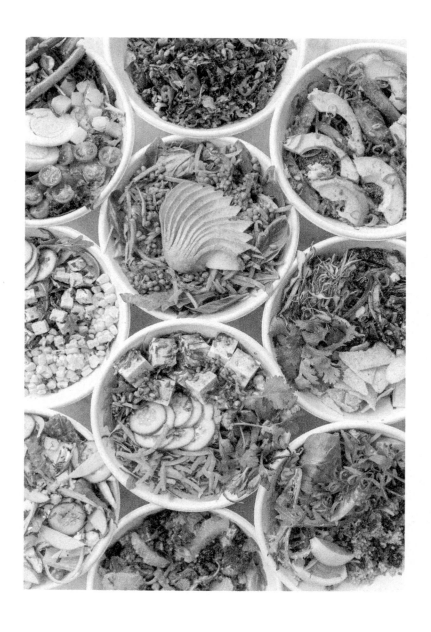

INTRODUCTION

Once upon a time, there was a young man named Thomas who had been suffering from Parkinson's disease for many years. He had tried various treatments, but nothing had worked. He was desperate for a cure.

One day, Thomas heard about a diet that could potentially help people with Parkinson's. He decided to give it a try and immediately began to follow the diet. He cut out all processed foods, sugar, dairy, and grains, and instead focused on eating whole, organic foods.

He soon began to feel better and within a few months, he was virtually symptom-free. He continued to follow the diet and eventually, his Parkinson's disease was completely cured.

Thomas was so excited that he had finally found a cure for his illness. He was able to lead a normal life again and was amazed at how much of a difference the right diet could make. He was so grateful for the opportunity to be free of his illness.

Thomas shared his story with everyone he could and spread the word about the power of a healthy diet.

He helped many others who were suffering from Parkinson's by advocating for the same diet that had cured him.

Thomas's story was a true testament to the power of a healthy diet and how it can change lives. He was an inspiration to many and his story will live on for generations.

Anti-Parkinson's drugs are drugs that are used to treat the symptoms of Parkinson's disease. Parkinson's disease is a progressive neurological disorder that affects the nerve cells in the brain that control movement.

The primary symptoms of Parkinson's disease are tremor, stiffness, and difficulty with coordination, balance, and walking. Although there is no cure for Parkinson's disease, anti-Parkinson's drugs can help to reduce symptoms and improve a person's quality of life.

Anti-Parkinson's drugs work by either increasing the amount of dopamine available in the brain or by mimicking the effects of dopamine. The neurotransmitter dopamine is in charge of regulating movement. By increasing the amount of dopamine available in the brain, anti-Parkinson's drugs can help to reduce tremor and stiffness, and improve coordination and balance.

There are several different types of anti-Parkinson's drugs available, including levodopa, dopamine agonists, anticholinergics, and MAO-B inhibitors. Levodopa is the most commonly prescribed anti-Parkinson's drug, and it works by increasing the amount of dopamine available in the brain.

Dopamine agonists, such as ropinirole and pramipexole, mimic the effects of dopamine in the brain. Anticholinergics, such as trihexyphenidyl, help to reduce muscle stiffness by blocking the action of a chemical called acetylcholine. MAO-B inhibitors, such as selegiline, help to slow the breakdown of dopamine in the brain.

In addition to medication, physical and occupational therapy can also be used to help reduce the symptoms of Parkinson's disease. Physical therapy can help to improve coordination, balance, and walking, while occupational therapy can help to improve daily living activities.

Other strategies, such as diet modification, exercise, and stress management, can also be used to help manage symptoms.

Although there is no cure for Parkinson's disease, anti-Parkinson's drugs, along with physical and occupational therapy and other lifestyle modifications, can help to reduce symptoms and improve a person's quality of life.

It is important to note that anti-Parkinson's drugs can have side effects, and it is important to discuss any potential side effects with your doctor before starting a new medication. Additionally, it is important to follow your doctor's instructions for taking your medication and to keep all follow-up appointments.

Overall, anti-Parkinson's drugs can be an effective treatment for Parkinson's disease, and when used in combination with other treatments and lifestyle modifications, can help to reduce symptoms and improve a person's quality of life.

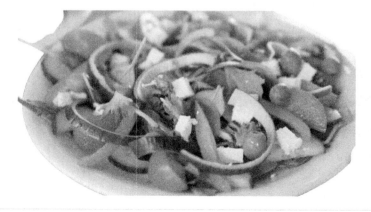

CHAPTER ONE

Anti-Parkinson Diet

Anti-Parkinson diets are special diets designed to reduce the symptoms of Parkinson's disease. They are highly individualized and should be tailored to the needs of each person.

There is no one-size-fits-all diet for Parkinson's, as everyone's dietary needs are different. However, there are some general principles that should be followed to ensure a nutritious, balanced diet.

First and foremost, it is important to get enough of the essential vitamins, minerals, and other nutrients needed to maintain good health. Varied, balanced diet rich in fruits, vegetables, whole grains, lean proteins, and healthy fats is recommended.

Eating enough of these foods can help to ensure that the body has the fuel it needs to function properly. In addition to eating a balanced diet, there are some specific foods that may be beneficial for people with Parkinson's.

Foods high in antioxidants, including blueberries, tomatoes, and spinach, may help to protect against cellular damage and reduce inflammation.

Omega-3 fatty acids found in fatty fish, flaxseeds, walnuts, and chia seeds may help to reduce the symptoms of Parkinson's. Certain B vitamins, including folate, B6, and B12, may be helpful in reducing the risk of developing Parkinson's or slowing its progression.

The importance of hydration should not be overlooked. Staying hydrated helps to keep the body functioning properly and can reduce the risk of developing complications related to Parkinson's. At least eight 8-ounce glasses of water should be consumed daily.

There are certain foods that may be beneficial to avoid as well. Caffeinated beverages, such as coffee and energy drinks, can cause tremors and other symptoms. Alcohol should also be avoided, as it can worsen some of the symptoms of Parkinson's.

Living with Parkinson's can be difficult, but with the right diet and lifestyle changes, it is possible to manage the symptoms and maintain a good quality of life.

An anti-Parkinson's diet is an important part of managing this condition and should be tailored to each individual's needs, an anti-Parkinson's diet is highly individualized and should be tailored to the needs of each person. Eating a balanced diet and getting enough of the essential vitamins, minerals, and other nutrients is important. Certain foods may be beneficial for people with Parkinson's, including those high in antioxidants, omega-3 fatty acids, and B vitamins. It is also important to stay hydrated and avoid certain foods that may worsen symptoms. With the right diet and lifestyle changes, it is possible to manage the symptoms and maintain a good quality of life.

Types of Parkinson's Diseases

Parkinson's disease is a progressive neurological disorder that affects movement and muscle control, caused by the death of a group of nerve cells in the part of the brain called the substantia nigra.

This leads to a lack of dopamine, a chemical in the brain responsible for controlling movement and coordination.

1. **Primary Parkinsonism:** This type of PD is caused by the death of dopamine-producing brain cells. It is the most common form of the disease and is typically treated with medications and lifestyle modifications.

2. **Secondary Parkinsonism:** This type of PD is caused by a medical condition or injury, such as a stroke or head trauma, that damages the brain. Treatment for this type of PD typically involves treating the underlying condition or injury.

3. **Atypical Parkinsonism:** This type of PD is caused by a genetic mutation or environmental toxin that affects the brain. Treatment for this type of PD may involve medications, lifestyle modifications, and other therapies.

4. **Drug-Induced Parkinsonism:** This type of PD is caused by certain medications, such as antipsychotics, that can interfere with brain function. Treatment for this type of PD typically involves stopping the medication and switching to a different drug.

5. **Vascular Parkinsonism:** This type of PD is caused by reduced blood flow to the brain, resulting in brain cell

damage. Treatment for this type of PD typically involves treating the underlying condition or injury.

6. Dementia with Lewy Bodies: This type of PD is caused by abnormal clumps of proteins in the brain called Lewy bodies. Treatment for this type of PD typically involves medications and lifestyle modifications.

7. Progressive Supranuclear Palsy: This type of PD is caused by damage to certain structures in the brain. Treatment for this type of PD typically involves medications and lifestyle modifications.

8. Multiple System Atrophy: This type of PD is caused by damage to certain structures in the brain. Treatment for this type of PD typically involves medications and lifestyle modifications.

9. Corticobasal Degeneration: This type of PD is caused by a genetic mutation that affects brain function. Treatment for this type of PD typically involves medications and lifestyle modifications.

10. Parkinsonism-Plus Syndromes: These types of PD are caused by various medical conditions or injuries that affect the brain. Treatment for this type of PD typically involves treating the underlying condition or injury.

11. Essential Tremor: This type of PD is caused by a genetic mutation that affects brain function.

Treatment for this type of PD typically involves medications, lifestyle modifications, and other therapies.

12. Postural Instability and Gait Disorders: This type of PD is caused by damage to certain structures in the brain. Treatment for this type of PD typically involves medications and lifestyle modifications.

13. Parkinson's Disease Dementia: This type of PD is caused by a progressive decline in cognitive function due to damage to certain structures in the brain. Treatment for this type of PD typically involves medications and lifestyle modifications.

14. Genetic Parkinsonism: This type of PD is caused by a genetic mutation that affects brain function. Treatment for this type of PD typically involves medications and lifestyle modifications.

15. Parkinson's Disease with Secondary Symptoms: This type of PD is caused by a combination of primary and secondary forms of PD.

Treatment for this type of PD typically involves medications and lifestyle modifications.

These types of PD can be caused by various medical conditions or injuries that affect the brain. Treatment for this type of PD typically involves treating the underlying condition or injury.

Parkinson's disease is a complex neurological disorder with a variety of causes and symptoms.

 Treatment for the various types of Parkinson's disease typically involves medications, lifestyle modifications, and other therapies depending on the underlying condition or injury.

Causes of Parkinson's Diseases

Parkinson's disease is a progressive neurological disorder. It's caused by a loss of nerve cells in the part of the brain that controls movement.

The primary symptoms of Parkinson's include tremor, slowness of movement, rigidity, and difficulties with balance and coordination.

1. Genetic: There is evidence that some forms of Parkinson's disease can be inherited. Mutations in several genes have been linked to the disorder, including SNCA, PARK2, and LRRK2.

2. Environmental: Exposure to environmental toxins such as pesticides and herbicides is believed to increase the risk of Parkinson's.

3. Aging: The risk of Parkinson's increases with age, although it can affect people of any age.

4. Neurotransmitter Imbalance: Imbalance of neurotransmitters, such as dopamine, is a known cause of Parkinson's disease.

5. Head Injury: Traumatic brain injury, including head trauma and stroke, can increase the risk of developing Parkinson's.

6. Viral Infection: Viral infections such as encephalitis have been linked to the development of Parkinson's.

7. Unknown Causes: In some cases, the cause of Parkinson's disease is unknown.

Parkinson's disease is a complex disorder with many possible causes. While some causes are known, the exact cause of the disorder remains unknown in many cases.

Symptoms of Parkinson's Disease

Parkinson's Disease is a neurological disorder that affects movement, causing tremors, rigidity and difficulty walking. Below are some of the common symptoms.

1. Tremor: A tremor, or shaking, usually begins in a limb, often your hands or fingers.

2. Rigidity: Stiffness or tension in the muscles can cause difficulty with movement and posture.

3. Bradykinesia: This is slowness of movement and difficulty initiating movement.

4. Postural Instability: This is difficulty maintaining balance, especially when turning or walking.

5. Gait Impairment: This can include shuffling steps, lack of arm swing, and a tendency to freeze while walking.

6. Loss of Automatic Movements: This can include blinking, smiling and swinging your arms as you walk.

7. Speech Changes: This can include slurring, monotonous speech and difficulty finding the right words.

8. Writing Changes: This can include a small, cramped handwriting known as micrographia.

9. Fatigue: This can include extreme tiredness and problems with sleeping.

10. Cognitive Impairment: This can include confusion, difficulty focusing and depression.

11. Loss of Sense of Smell: This is often an early symptom of Parkinson's Disease.

12. Constipation: This can be a symptom of Parkinson's Disease due to the slowing of the digestive system.

13. Unexplained Pain: This can include persistent pain, stiffness and cramping.

Ways to Prevent Parkinson's Diseases

Parkinson's disease is a degenerative neurological condition that impairs movement.

It is a degenerative disorder caused by the gradual loss of dopamine-producing cells in the brain. It is characterized by tremors, stiffness, and slowed movement.

Although there is no known cure for Parkinson's disease, there are ways to help slow the progression and reduce symptoms. Here are some tips on how to prevent Parkinson's disease.

1. Exercise: Regular physical activity helps reduce the risk of Parkinson's disease and improve overall health. Exercise can help increase dopamine production, improve balance and coordination, and reduce stress.

2. Maintain a Healthy Diet: Eating a healthy diet can help reduce the risk of developing Parkinson's disease. A balanced diet that includes plenty of fruits, vegetables, whole grains, and lean proteins can help protect against diseases like Parkinson's.

3. Avoid Toxins: Avoiding toxins, such as pesticides and herbicides, can help reduce the risk of Parkinson's disease.

4. Get Enough Sleep: Getting enough sleep can help protect against Parkinson's disease.

Lack of sleep can increase oxidative stress, which can damage the brain and increase the risk of Parkinson's.

5. Reduce Stress: Reducing stress can help lower the risk of Parkinson's disease. Stress can increase inflammation and oxidative stress, which can damage the brain and increase the risk of Parkinson's disease.

6. Limit Alcohol Consumption: Limiting alcohol intake can reduce the risk of Parkinson's disease. Heavy drinking can increase oxidative stress and damage the brain, which can increase the risk of Parkinson's disease.

7. Take Dietary Supplements: Taking dietary supplements, such as omega-3 fatty acids, vitamin B6, and CoenzymeQ10, can help reduce the risk of Parkinson's disease.

These tips can help reduce the risk of developing Parkinson's disease.

However, it is important to consult with your doctor before taking any new supplements or beginning any new exercise program.

Overall, Parkinson's disease is a serious disorder that can cause debilitating symptoms. While there is no known cure, there are ways to help slow the progression and reduce symptoms.

Following these tips can help reduce the risk of developing Parkinson's disease and help improve overall health.

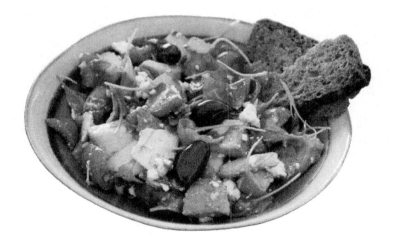

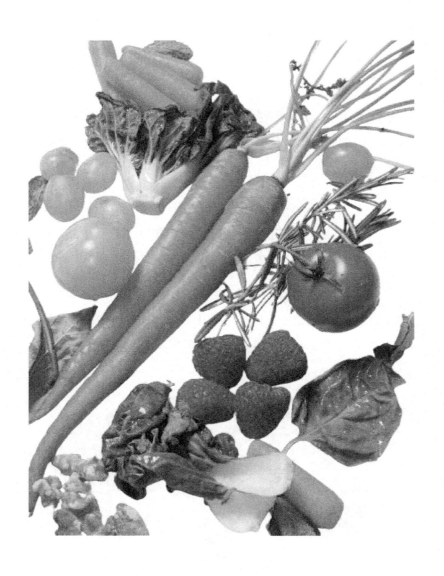

CHAPTER TWO

Anti-Parkinson's Diet and Benefits

Parkinson's disease is a chronic and progressive movement disorder that affects an estimated one million Americans and more than 10 million people worldwide. It is caused by the death of dopamine-producing brain cells, leading to impaired movement, loss of coordination, and other symptoms such as tremors, stiffness, and difficulty with balance.

While there is no cure for Parkinson's, there are treatments that can help manage symptoms, including medications, therapies, and lifestyle changes, such as following an Anti-Parkinson's diet.

An Anti-Parkinson's diet is an eating plan that is tailored to the needs of individuals with Parkinson's disease. It focuses on providing nutrients that can support optimal brain health and help improve symptoms, as well as reduce the risk of other health problems.

While there is no "one-size-fits-all" diet for Parkinson's, there are some general principles that can be followed.

The first principle is to eat a balanced diet that is rich in fresh fruits and vegetables, whole grains, lean proteins, and healthy fats. Eating a variety of nutrient-dense foods is important for maintaining overall health and managing Parkinson's symptoms. Fruits, vegetables, and whole grains are especially important, as they are packed with antioxidants and other essential vitamins and minerals. Eating a diet rich in these foods can help protect against cell damage, reduce inflammation, and improve overall brain health.

The second principle of an Anti-Parkinson's diet is to ensure adequate hydration. Drinking enough water is essential for proper brain function and overall health. People with Parkinson's may need to drink more water than average, as dehydration can worsen symptoms.

The third principle is to limit processed foods. Processed foods tend to be high in sugar, salt, fat, and other unhealthy ingredients, which can contribute to inflammation and worsen symptoms.

Eating a diet that is low in processed foods can help reduce inflammation and improve overall health.

Finally, it is important to get regular exercise. Maintaining good physical and mental health requires regular exercise. Moving the body and engaging in physical activity can help reduce stiffness and improve coordination, as well as release endorphins that provide a sense of well-being.

Following an anti-Parkinson's diet and leading an active lifestyle can help improve symptoms and reduce the risk of other health problems.

Eating a balanced diet that is rich in fresh fruits and vegetables, whole grains, lean proteins, and healthy fats, as well as drinking enough water and limiting processed foods, can help protect against cell damage, reduce inflammation, and improve overall health.

Additionally, getting regular exercise can help reduce stiffness, improve coordination, and provide a sense of well-being. By following these principles, individuals with Parkinson's can improve their quality of life and better manage their symptoms.

How to Follow an Anti-Parkinson's Diet

Millions of people worldwide are afflicted by the crippling neurological illness known as Parkinson's disease. While there is no known cure, some treatments can help reduce symptoms and improve quality of life. One such treatment is following a healthy diet, which can help slow down the progression of the disease and provide vital nutrients to the body. A Parkinson's diet should include foods that are high in essential vitamins and minerals, as well as those that are low in saturated fats and processed sugars. In this article, we will provide a comprehensive guide for following an anti-Parkinson's diet, including what foods to eat and what foods to avoid.

What is an Anti-Parkinson's Diet?

An anti-Parkinson's diet is a dietary plan specifically designed to reduce the symptoms of Parkinson's disease. It should include foods that are high in essential vitamins and minerals, such as B-vitamins, omega-3 fatty acids, and antioxidants.

These nutrients can help protect the neurons in the brain, which can slow the progression of the disease.

Additionally, an anti-Parkinson's diet should limit the intake of saturated fats and processed sugars, as these can raise blood sugar levels and cause inflammation, both of which can exacerbate Parkinson's symptoms.

What Foods Should You Eat?

• **Fruits and Vegetables:** Eating a variety of fresh fruits and vegetables is essential for any healthy diet, but especially for those with Parkinson's.

Fruits and vegetables are packed with vitamins, minerals, and antioxidants, which can help protect the brain and reduce inflammation.

• **Lean Protein:** Eating lean proteins, such as poultry, fish, and beans, can help provide the body with essential amino acids. These proteins can help reduce inflammation and provide the body with essential nutrients.

• **Whole Grains:** Eating whole grains, such as quinoa, oats, and brown rice, can help provide the body with fiber and B-vitamins. These can help reduce inflammation and improve digestion.

• **Healthy Fats:** Eating healthy fats, such as avocados, nuts, and seeds, can help provide the body with essential omega-3 fatty acids.

These can help reduce inflammation and improve neurological functioning.

• **Herbs and Spices:** Eating herbs and spices, such as turmeric and ginger, can help reduce inflammation and provide the body with antioxidants.

What Foods Should You Avoid?

• **Processed Foods**: Processed foods, such as chips, cookies, and candy, should be avoided as they are high in saturated fats, processed sugars, and preservatives, all of which can raise blood sugar levels and cause inflammation.

• **Refined Carbohydrates**: Refined carbohydrates, such as white bread and pasta, should be avoided as they are low in essential vitamins and minerals and can raise blood sugar levels.

• **High-Fat Dairy:** High-fat dairy, such as whole milk and cheese, should be avoided as they are high in saturated fats, which can raise blood sugar levels and cause inflammation.

• **Fried Foods:** Fried foods, such as French fries and doughnuts, should be avoided as they are high in saturated fats and processed sugars, both of which can raise blood sugar levels and cause inflammation.

Following an anti-Parkinson's diet can be a great way to reduce symptoms and improve quality of life for those with the disease. By focusing on eating fresh, whole foods that are high in essential vitamins and minerals, as well as limiting the intake of saturated fats and processed sugars, those with Parkinson's can improve their overall health and help slow down the progression of the disease.

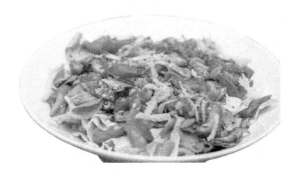

7 days Anti-Parkinson Diet

Day 1

1. Breakfast: Overnight Oats with Blueberries

Ingredients:

- 1/2 cup rolled oats

- 1/3 cup milk

- 1/4 cup plain Greek yogurt

- 1/4 teaspoon ground cinnamon

- 1/4 cup blueberries

Instructions:

1. In a bowl combine oats, milk, yogurt, and cinnamon.

2. Mix well, then add blueberries.

3. Cover and refrigerate overnight.

4. Enjoy the next morning!

2. Lunch: Quinoa and Kale Salad

Ingredients:

- 1 cup cooked quinoa

- 2 cups chopped kale

- 1/2 cup sliced carrots

- 1/2 cup diced red bell pepper

- 1/4 cup chopped walnuts

- 2 tablespoons olive oil

- 2 tablespoons lemon juice

- 1 teaspoon honey

- Salt and pepper to taste

Instructions:

1. In a bowl, mix together quinoa, kale, carrots, bell pepper, and walnuts.

2. In a separate bowl, whisk together olive oil, lemon juice, honey, salt, and pepper.

3. Pour the dressing over the quinoa and kale mixture and toss to combine.

4. Serve chilled.

3. Dinner: Baked Salmon with Spinach

Ingredients:

• 2 salmon fillets

• 2 tablespoons olive oil

• 2 cloves garlic, minced

• 1 teaspoon dried oregano

• Salt and pepper to taste

• 2 cups baby spinach

Instructions:

1. Preheat oven to 350°F.

2. Salmon fillets should be placed in a baking dish.

3. Drizzle with olive oil and sprinkle with garlic, oregano, salt, and pepper.

4. Bake for 15 minutes.

5. Add spinach to the baking dish and bake for another 5 minutes.

6. Serve warm.

Day 2

1. Breakfast: Avocado Toast with Egg

Ingredients:

• 2 slices whole wheat bread

• 1/2 avocado, mashed

• 1/2 teaspoon ground cumin

• 1/4 teaspoon garlic powder

• 1 egg

• Salt and pepper to taste

Instructions:

1. Toast bread slices in a toaster.

2. Spread mashed avocado on toast and sprinkle with cumin and garlic powder.

3. Fry egg in a skillet over medium heat until desired doneness.

4. Place egg on top of avocado toast and season with salt and pepper.

5. Enjoy!

2. Lunch: Chickpea and Spinach Curry

Ingredients:

• 2 tablespoons olive oil

• 1 onion, diced

• 2 cloves garlic, minced

• 2 teaspoons curry powder

• 1 teaspoon ground cumin

• 1/2 teaspoon ground coriander

• 1 (14-ounce) can diced tomatoes

• 1 (15-ounce) can of washed and drained chickpeas

• 2 cups baby spinach

• Salt and pepper to taste

Instructions:

1. In a big skillet, heat the oil over medium heat.

2. Add the onion and garlic and simmer for about 5 minutes, or until tender.

3. Add curry powder, cumin, and coriander and cook for 1 minute.

4. Add tomatoes and chickpeas and simmer for 10 minutes.

5. Stir in spinach and season with salt and pepper.

6. Serve over cooked brown rice.

3. Dinner: Lentil Soup with Vegetables

Ingredients:

• 2 tablespoons olive oil

• 1 onion, diced

• 2 cloves garlic, minced

• 1 carrot, diced

• 1 celery stalk, diced

• 1 (15-ounce) can of washed and drained lentils

- 4 cups vegetable broth

- 1 teaspoon dried oregano

- 1 teaspoon dried thyme

- Salt and pepper to taste

Instructions:

1. In a big pot, heat the oil over medium heat.

2. Include the onion, garlic, carrot, and celery and simmer for about 5 minutes, or until softened.

3. Bring to a boil the lentils, stock, oregano, and thyme.

4. Lower the heat to low and let the pot simmer for 15 minutes.

5. Season with salt and pepper and serve.

Day 3

1. Breakfast: Yogurt Parfait with Berries

Ingredients:

- 1/2 cup plain Greek yogurt

- 1/4 cup granola

- 1/4 cup fresh berries

- 1 tablespoon honey

Instructions:

1. In a bowl, layer yogurt, granola, and berries.

2. Drizzle with honey and enjoy!

2. Lunch: Kale, Apple, and Almond Salad

Ingredients:

- 2 cups chopped kale

- 1/2 apple, diced

- 1/4 cup sliced almonds

- 2 tablespoons olive oil

- 1 tablespoon lemon juice

- 1 teaspoon Dijon mustard

- Salt and pepper to taste

Instructions:

1. In a bowl, mix together kale, apple, and almonds.

2. In a separate bowl, whisk together olive oil, lemon juice, mustard, salt, and pepper.

3. Pour the dressing over the kale mixture and toss to combine.

4. Serve chilled.

3. Dinner: Baked Chicken with Roasted Vegetables

Ingredients:

• 2 chicken breasts

• 2 tablespoons olive oil

• 1 teaspoon garlic powder

• 1 teaspoon dried oregano

• 1/2 teaspoon dried thyme

• Salt and pepper to taste

• 2 cups chopped vegetables (e.g., carrots, potatoes, bell peppers)

Instructions:

1. Preheat oven to 375°F.

2. Put chicken breasts in a baking dish.

3. Drizzle with olive oil and sprinkle with garlic powder, oregano, thyme, salt, and pepper.

4. Place vegetables around the chicken.

5. Bake for 25 minutes.

6. Serve warm.

Day 4

1. Breakfast: Smoothie Bowl

Ingredients:

- 1/2 cup frozen pineapple

- 1/2 banana

- 1/2 cup plain Greek yogurt

- 1/4 cup milk

- 1 tablespoon honey

• Toppings: chia seeds, sliced almonds, coconut flakes

Instructions:

1. Place pineapple, banana, yogurt, milk, and honey in a blender.

2. Blend until smooth.

3. Pour into a bowl and top with desired toppings.

4. Enjoy!

2. Lunch: Bean and Avocado Burritos

Ingredients:

• 2 whole wheat tortillas

• 1/2 cup cooked black beans

• 1/2 avocado, sliced

• 1/4 cup diced tomatoes

• 1/4 cup shredded cheese

• 2 tablespoons chopped fresh cilantro

• Salt and pepper to taste

Instructions:

1. Place tortillas on a plate.

2. Top each tortilla with beans, avocado, tomatoes, cheese, and cilantro.

3. Season with salt and pepper.

4. Fold tortillas and enjoy!

3. Dinner: Stuffed Peppers

Ingredients:

• 4 bell peppers, halved and seeded

• 1 cup cooked quinoa

• 1/2 cup diced tomatoes

• 1/4 cup chopped olives

• 2 tablespoons chopped fresh parsley

• 2 tablespoons olive oil

• 2 cloves garlic, minced

• Salt and pepper to taste

Instructions:

1. Preheat oven to 375°F.

2. Place bell peppers in a baking dish.

3. In a bowl, mix together quinoa, tomatoes, olives, parsley, olive oil, garlic, salt, and pepper.

4. Fill each pepper half with quinoa mixture.

5. Bake for 25 minutes.

6. Serve warm.

Day 5

1. Breakfast: Omelet with Mushrooms and Spinach

Ingredients:

• 2 eggs

• 2 tablespoons milk

• 1/4 cup sliced mushrooms

• 1/4 cup chopped spinach

• 2 tablespoons shredded cheese

- 1 tablespoon olive oil

- Salt and pepper to taste

Instructions:

2. In a skillet, heat the oil over medium heat.

3. Include the mushrooms and spinach and simmer for 5 minutes or until spinach is tender.

4. When the eggs are nearly set, pour the egg mixture into the skillet.

5. Cheese is sprinkled on top, then salt and pepper are added.

6. Fold omelet in half and cook for another minute.

7. Serve warm.

2. Lunch: Roasted Root Vegetables

Ingredients:

- 1 sweet potato, cubed

- 1 parsnip, cubed

- 1 turnip, cubed

- 1 tablespoon olive oil

- 1 teaspoon dried rosemary

- Salt and pepper to taste

Instructions:

1. Preheat oven to 375°F.

2. Place sweet potato, parsnip, and turnip on a baking sheet.

3. Drizzle with olive oil and season with rosemary, salt, and pepper.

4. Roast for 25 minutes.

5. Serve warm.

3. Dinner: Lentil and Sweet Potato Stew

Ingredients:

- 2 tablespoons olive oil

- 1 onion, diced

- 2 cloves garlic, minced

- 1 teaspoon ground cumin

- 2 cups vegetable broth

- 1 (15-ounce) can lentils, drained and rinsed

- 1 sweet potato, cubed

- 1/2 cup chopped kale

- Salt and pepper to taste

Instructions:

1. In a big pot, heat the oil over medium heat.

2. Add the onion and garlic and simmer for about 5 minutes, or until tender.

3. Bring to a boil the cumin, broth, lentils, and sweet potato.

4. Lower the heat to low and let the pot simmer for 15 minutes.

5. Stir in kale and season with salt and pepper.

6. Serve warm.

Day 6

1. Breakfast: Banana and Walnut Oatmeal

Ingredients:

- 1/2 cup rolled oats

- 1/3 cup milk

- 1/2 banana, mashed

- 2 tablespoons chopped walnuts

- 1 tablespoon honey

- 1/4 teaspoon ground cinnamon

Instructions:

1. In a small pot, combine oats, milk, banana, and walnuts.

2. Cook over medium heat until oats are soft and creamy, about 5 minutes.

3. Stir in honey and cinnamon.

4. Serve warm.

2. Lunch: Avocado and Chickpea Wrap

Ingredients:

- 2 whole wheat tortillas

- 1/2 avocado, mashed

- 1/2 cup cooked chickpeas

- 2 tablespoons diced tomatoes

• 2 tablespoons chopped fresh cilantro

• 1 tablespoon lime juice

• Salt and pepper to taste

Instructions:

1. Place tortillas on a plate.

2. Spread mashed avocado on each tortilla.

3. Top with chickpeas, tomatoes, cilantro, lime juice, salt, and pepper.

4. Fold tortillas and enjoy!

3. Dinner: Baked Tilapia with Roasted Broccoli

Ingredients:

• 2 tilapia fillets

• 2 tablespoons olive oil

• 1 teaspoon garlic powder

• 1 teaspoon dried oregano

• 2 cups broccoli florets

• Salt and pepper to taste

Instructions:

1. Preheat oven to 375°F.

2. Place tilapia fillets in a baking dish.

3. Drizzle with olive oil and sprinkle with garlic powder, oregano, salt, and pepper.

4. Place broccoli florets around the tilapia.

5. Bake for 15 minutes.

6. Serve warm.

Day 7

1. Breakfast: Banana-Almond Smoothie

Ingredients:

• 1 banana

• 1/2 cup plain Greek yogurt

• 1/4 cup milk

• 1 tablespoon almond butter

• 1 teaspoon honey

Instructions:

1. Place banana, yogurt, milk, almond butter, and honey in a blender.

2. Blend until smooth.

3. Pour into a glass and enjoy!

2. Lunch: Quinoa and Vegetable Salad

Ingredients:

• 1 cup cooked quinoa

• 1/2 cup diced cucumber

• 1/2 cup diced tomatoes

• 1/4 cup diced red onion

• 2 tablespoons chopped fresh parsley

• 2 tablespoons olive oil

• 2 tablespoons lemon juice

• Salt and pepper to taste

Instructions:

1. In a bowl, mix together quinoa, cucumber, tomatoes, red onion, and parsley.

2. In a separate bowl, whisk together olive oil, lemon juice, salt, and pepper.

3. Pour the dressing over the quinoa mixture and toss to combine.

4. Serve chilled.

3. Dinner: Baked Salmon with Asparagus

Ingredients:

• 2 salmon fillets

• 2 tablespoons olive oil

• 2 cloves garlic, minced

• 1 teaspoon dried oregano

• Salt and pepper to taste

• 1 bunch asparagus, trimmed

Instructions:

1. Preheat oven to 350°F.

2. Salmon fillets should be placed in a baking dish.

3. Drizzle with olive oil and sprinkle with garlic, oregano, salt, and pepper.

4. Place asparagus around the salmon.

5. Bake for 15 minutes.

6. Serve warm.

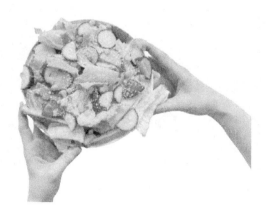

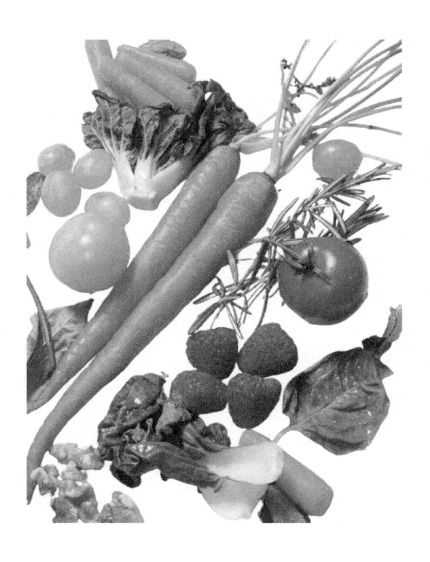

CHAPTER THREE

Anti-Parkinson's Diet Breakfast Recipes

1. Overnight Oats with Berries

Start your day with a healthy and nutritious breakfast that is packed with antioxidants from the berries. This recipe takes 10 minutes to prepare and can be made ahead of time for convenience.

Ingredients:

- 1 cup oats

- 2 cups almond milk

- 1 tablespoon honey

- 1 teaspoon cinnamon

- 1/4 teaspoon nutmeg

- 1/2 cup frozen berries

Instructions:

1. In a medium bowl, combine the oats, almond milk, honey, cinnamon, and nutmeg.

2. Stir until ingredients are evenly combined.

3. Pour the mixture into a mason jar or airtight container.

4. Add the frozen berries and stir until evenly distributed.

5. Place in the refrigerator overnight.

6. Enjoy the next morning!

Cooking Time: 10 minutes (plus overnight refrigeration)

2. Banana-Blueberry Smoothie Bowl

Start your day with a creamy and delicious smoothie bowl that is full of natural sweetness from the bananas and blueberries.

This recipe takes only 5 minutes to prepare.

Ingredients:

- 1 frozen banana

- 1/2 cup frozen blueberries

- 1/4 cup almond milk

- 1/4 teaspoon ground cinnamon

- 1 tablespoon chia seeds

Instructions:

1. In a blender, combine the banana, blueberries, almond milk, and cinnamon.

2. Continue blending until the mixture has a smooth and creamy texture.

3. Pour the mixture into a bowl.

4. Sprinkle the chia seeds on top and stir until evenly distributed.

5. Enjoy immediately!

Cooking Time: 5 minutes

3. Egg, Spinach, and Tomato Breakfast Burrito

Start your day with a flavourful and protein-packed breakfast burrito. It simply takes ten minutes to prepare this recipe.

Ingredients:

- 4 eggs

- 1/4 cup shredded cheese

- 1/2 cup cooked spinach

- 1/2 cup diced tomatoes

- 4 whole wheat tortillas

- 2 tablespoons olive oil

Instructions:

1. In a medium bowl, whisk together the eggs and cheese.

2. In a big skillet over medium heat, warm the olive oil.

3. Add the egg mixture and cook until the eggs are set, stirring occasionally.

4. Remove from heat and stir in the spinach and tomatoes.

5. Lay out the tortillas and divide the egg mixture among them.

6. Roll up the tortillas and enjoy!

Cooking Time: 10 minutes

4. Avocado Toast with Feta and Tomatoes

Start your day with a delicious and savoury breakfast that is full of healthy fats from the avocado and feta. This recipe takes only 5 minutes to prepare.

Ingredients:

- 2 slices of whole wheat bread

- 1 avocado

- 1/4 cup feta cheese

- 1/4 cup diced tomatoes

- 2 tablespoons olive oil

Instructions:

1. Toast the bread in a toaster or in a skillet over medium heat until golden brown.

2. While the bread is toasting, mash the avocado in a small bowl.

3. Cover the toast with the mashed avocado.

4. Sprinkle the feta cheese and diced tomatoes on top.

5. Drizzle with olive oil and enjoy!

Cooking Time: 5 minutes

5. Baked Oatmeal with Apples and Walnuts

Start your day with a wholesome and comforting breakfast that is full of fibber and healthy fats. It simply takes thirty minutes to prepare this recipe.

Ingredients:

- 2 cups rolled oats

- 2 cups almond milk

- 2 tablespoons honey

- 1 teaspoon cinnamon

- 1/4 teaspoon nutmeg

- 1 apple, diced

- 1/4 cup walnuts, chopped

Instructions:

1. Preheat oven to 350°F.

2. In a medium bowl, combine the oats, almond milk, honey, cinnamon, and nutmeg.

3. Stir until ingredients are evenly combined.

4. Grease an 8-inch baking dish with cooking spray.

5. Pour the oat mixture into the dish and spread it evenly.

6. Top with the diced apples and chopped walnuts.

7. Bake for 30 minutes.

8. Enjoy warm!

Cooking Time: 30 minutes

6. Greek Yogurt Parfait with Berries and Granola

Start your day with a light and refreshing breakfast that is full of protein and antioxidants. This recipe takes only 5 minutes to prepare.

Ingredients:

- 1 cup Greek yogurt

- 1/2 cup frozen berries

- 1/4 cup granola

- 1 tablespoon honey

Instructions:

1. In a medium bowl, combine the Greek yogurt, berries, and granola.

2. Stir until ingredients are evenly combined.

3. Pour the mixture into a glass or bowl.

4. Drizzle with honey and enjoy!

Cooking Time: 5 minutes

7. Breakfast Quinoa Bowl

Start your day with a hearty and satisfying breakfast that is full of fiber and protein. It simply takes ten minutes to prepare this recipe.

Ingredients:

- 1/2 cup quinoa

- 1 cup almond milk

- 1 teaspoon cinnamon

- 1/4 teaspoon nutmeg

- 1/4 cup raisins

- 1/4 cup walnuts, chopped

- 2 tablespoons honey

Instructions:

1. In a medium saucepan, bring the quinoa and almond milk to a boil.

2. Reduce heat to low and simmer, stirring occasionally, until the quinoa is cooked and the liquid has been absorbed, about 10 minutes.

3. Meanwhile, in a small bowl, combine the cinnamon, nutmeg, raisins, and walnuts.

4. Once the quinoa is cooked, stir in the cinnamon mixture.

5. Drizzle with honey and enjoy!

Cooking Time: 10 minutes

8. Savory Oatmeal with Mushrooms and Spinach

Start your day with a warm and comforting breakfast that is full of flavor. It simply takes fifteen minutes to prepare this recipe.

Ingredients:

- 1 cup oats

- 2 cups vegetable broth

- 1/2 teaspoon garlic powder

- 1/2 teaspoon onion powder

- 1/4 teaspoon black pepper

- 1/4 cup mushrooms, chopped

- 1/4 cup cooked spinach

- 2 tablespoons olive oil

Instructions:

1. In a medium saucepan, combine the oats, vegetable broth, garlic powder, onion powder, and black pepper.

2. Bring to a boil, then reduce heat to low and simmer, stirring occasionally, until the oats are cooked and the liquid has been absorbed, about 10 minutes.

3. Heat the olive oil in a small skillet over medium heat.

4. Add the mushrooms and cook until softened, about 5 minutes.

5. Add the cooked spinach and stir until combined.

6. Add the mushroom and spinach mixture to the cooked oatmeal and stir until evenly combined.

7. Enjoy warm!

Cooking Time: 15 minutes

9. Peanut Butter and Banana Toast

Start your day with a tasty and satisfying breakfast that is full of healthy fats and natural sweetness. It simply takes five minutes to prepare this recipe.

Ingredients:

- 2 slices of whole wheat bread

- 2 tablespoons peanut butter

- 1 banana, sliced

- 1 tablespoon honey

Instructions:

1. Toast the bread in a toaster or in a skillet over medium heat until golden brown.

2. Spread the peanut butter on the toast.

3. Top with the banana slices and drizzle with honey.

4. Enjoy immediately!

Cooking Time: 5 minutes

10. Omelet with Asparagus and Cheese

Start your day with a flavorful and protein-packed omelet. It simply takes ten minutes to prepare this recipe.

Ingredients:

- 4 eggs

- 1/4 cup shredded cheese

- 1/2 cup cooked asparagus

- 2 tablespoons olive oil

Instructions:

1. In a medium bowl, whisk together the eggs and cheese.

2. In a big skillet over medium heat, warm the olive oil.

3. Add the egg mixture and cook until the eggs are set, stirring occasionally.

4. Add the cooked asparagus and stir until evenly distributed.

5. Flip the omelet and cook until it is golden brown.

6. Enjoy warm!

Cooking Time: 10 minutes

Anti-Parkinson's Diet Lunch Recipes

1. Lentil and Vegetable Soup

This high-fiber and heart-healthy soup is packed with protein and vitamins and minerals. It takes about 25 minutes to make, making it an easy and nutritious lunch.

Ingredients:

- 2 tablespoons olive oil

- 1 onion, chopped

- 2 cloves garlic, minced

- 1 cup dry lentils, rinsed

- 1 teaspoon ground cumin

- 1 teaspoon dried oregano

- 4 cups vegetable broth

- 1 large carrot, diced

- 1 large celery stalk, diced

- 1 medium zucchini, diced

- 1 teaspoon sea salt

- 1/4 teaspoon freshly ground black pepper

Instructions:

1. In a big pot over medium heat, warm the olive oil.

2. Include the onion and garlic and sauté for about 5 minutes, or until the onion is transparent.

3. Add the lentils, cumin, and oregano and stir to combine.

4. Add the vegetable broth, carrot, celery, and zucchini.

5. Bring to a boil, reduce heat to low, and simmer for 15-20 minutes, or until the lentils are tender.

6. Add salt and pepper to taste before serving.

Cooking Time: 25 minutes

2. Quinoa Salad

This protein-packed salad is perfect for a healthy and flavorful lunch. It takes about 20 minutes to make.

Ingredients:

- 1 cup quinoa, rinsed

- 2 cups water

- 1 tablespoon olive oil

- 2 cloves garlic, minced

- 1 red bell pepper, diced

- 1/2 cup frozen corn, thawed

- 1/2 cup washed and drained canned black beans

- 2 tablespoons fresh cilantro, chopped

- 2 tablespoons fresh lime juice

- 1/4 teaspoon sea salt

- 1/4 teaspoon freshly ground black pepper

Instructions:

1. Bring the quinoa and water to a boil in a medium pot.

2. Reduce heat to low, cover, and simmer for 15 minutes, or until the quinoa is tender and the water is absorbed.

3. In a big skillet over medium heat, warm the olive oil.

4. Add the garlic, bell pepper, and corn and sauté for 5 minutes, or until the vegetables are tender.

5. Add the black beans and cooked quinoa and stir to combine.

6. Remove from heat and stir in the cilantro, lime juice, salt, and pepper.

7. Serve warm or cold.

Cooking Time: 20 minutes

3. Hummus and Vegetable Wrap

This wrap is an easy and delicious lunch that packs a punch of flavor.

It takes about 10 minutes to make.

Ingredients:

- 2 whole wheat or gluten-free tortillas

- 1/4 cup hummus

- 1/2 cup shredded carrots

- 1/2 cup shredded cabbage

- 1/4 cup diced tomatoes

- 2 tablespoons chopped fresh parsley

Instructions:

1. Spread the hummus onto each tortilla.

2. Top with the shredded carrots, cabbage, tomatoes, and parsley.

3. Wrap the tortillas in a roll, and then fasten with a toothpick.

4. Cut each wrap in half and serve.

Cooking Time: 10 minutes

4. Avocado Toast

Avocado toast is light and refreshing, making it a perfect lunch. It takes about 5 minutes to make.

Ingredients:

- 2 slices whole wheat or gluten-free bread

- 1 ripe avocado

- Juice of 1/2 lemon

- 1/4 teaspoon sea salt

- 1/4 teaspoon freshly ground black pepper

Instructions:

1. Toast the bread.

2. Cut the avocado in half and remove the pit.

3. Scoop out the avocado and mash in a bowl.

4. Add the salt, pepper, and lemon juice.

5. Spread the avocado mixture onto the toast and serve.

Cooking Time: 5 minutes

5. Lentil and Kale Salad

This salad is a nutritional powerhouse and takes about 25 minutes to make.

Ingredients:

- 1 cup dry lentils, rinsed

- 2 cups water

- 2 tablespoons olive oil

- 2 cloves garlic, minced

- 1/2 teaspoon sea salt

- 1/4 teaspoon freshly ground black pepper

- 4 cups kale, chopped

- 1/2 cup chopped tomatoes

- 1/4 cup crumbled feta cheese

- 2 tablespoons fresh lemon juice

Instructions:

1. Bring the lentils and water to a boil in a medium pot.

2. Reduce heat to low, cover, and simmer for 15 minutes, or until the lentils are tender and the water is absorbed.

3. In a big skillet over medium heat, warm the olive oil.

4. Add the garlic, salt, and pepper and sauté for 1 minute.

5. Add the kale and sauté for 5 minutes, or until the kale is wilted.

6. Add the cooked lentils and tomatoes and stir to combine.

7. Remove from heat and stir in the feta cheese and lemon juice.

8. Serve warm or cold.

Cooking Time: 25 minutes

6. Tofu and Veggie Stir Fry

This stir fry is packed with flavor and only takes about 20 minutes to make.

Ingredients:

- 1 tablespoon sesame oil

- 1 box cubed, drained extra-firm tofu

- 1/2 teaspoon sea salt

- 1/4 teaspoon freshly ground black pepper

- 1/2 cup carrots, sliced

- 1/2 cup bell pepper, diced

- 1/2 cup snap peas

- 1/2 cup mushrooms, sliced

- 2 cloves garlic, minced

- 2 tablespoons soy sauce

Instructions:

3. In a big skillet over medium heat, warm the sesame oil.

2. Add the tofu, salt, and pepper and cook for 5 minutes, or until the tofu is golden brown.

3. Add the carrots, bell pepper, snap peas, mushrooms, and garlic and sauté for 5 minutes, or until the vegetables are tender.

4. Add the soy sauce and stir to combine.

5. Serve warm.

Cooking Time: 20 minutes

7. Roasted Vegetable Sandwich

This sandwich is easy to make and loaded with flavor.

It takes about 20 minutes to prepare.

Ingredients:

- 2 tablespoons olive oil

- 1 large sweet potato, cubed

- 1 large red bell pepper, diced

- 1 large yellow onion, diced

- 1 teaspoon dried oregano

- 1 teaspoon sea salt

- 1/4 teaspoon freshly ground black pepper

- 4 slices whole wheat or gluten-free bread

- 2 tablespoons hummus

- 2 tablespoons Dijon mustard

Instructions:

1. Preheat oven to 375°F.

2. Toss the sweet potato, bell pepper, and onion with the olive oil, oregano, salt, and pepper.

3. Spread the vegetables onto a baking sheet and roast for 15 minutes, or until the vegetables are tender.

4. Toast the bread.

5. Spread the hummus and Dijon mustard onto each slice of toast.

6. Top with the roasted vegetables and serve.

Cooking Time: 20 minutes

8. Chickpea Salad Sandwich

This protein-packed sandwich is perfect for an easy and healthy lunch. It takes about 10 minutes to prepare.

Ingredients:

- 1 can chickpeas, drained and rinsed

- 2 tablespoons olive oil

- 2 tablespoons fresh lemon juice

- 1/4 teaspoon sea salt

- 1/4 teaspoon freshly ground black pepper

- 4 slices whole wheat or gluten-free bread

- 2 tablespoons hummus

- 2 tablespoons chopped fresh parsley

Instructions:

1. Mash the chickpeas in a bowl.

2. Stir in the olive oil, lemon juice, salt, and pepper.

3. Toast the bread.

4. Spread the hummus onto each slice of toast.

5. Top with the chickpea mixture and sprinkle with the parsley.

6. Serve.

Cooking Time: 10 minutes

9. Lentil and Spinach Wrap

This wrap is packed with protein, fiber, and vitamins and minerals. It takes about 10 minutes to prepare.

Ingredients:

- 2 whole wheat or gluten-free tortillas

- 1 cup cooked lentils

- 2 cups baby spinach

- 1/4 cup feta cheese, crumbled

- 2 tablespoons fresh lemon juice

Instructions:

1. Spread the lentils onto each tortilla.

2. Top with the spinach, feta cheese, and lemon juice.

3. Wrap the tortillas in a roll, and then fasten with a toothpick.

4. To serve, divide each wrap in half.

Cooking Time: 10 minutes

10. Avocado and Tomato Sandwich

This sandwich is quick and easy to make and packs a punch of flavor. It takes about 10 minutes to prepare.

Ingredients:

- 2 slices of gluten-free or whole wheat bread

- 1 ripe avocado

- Juice of 1/2 lemon

- 1/4 teaspoon sea salt

- 1/4 teaspoon freshly ground black pepper

- 2 tablespoons hummus

- 1 medium tomato, sliced

Instructions:

1. Toast the bread.

2. Cut the avocado in half and remove the pit.

3. Scoop out the avocado and mash in a bowl.

4. Add the salt, pepper, and lemon juice.

5. Spread the hummus onto each slice of toast.

6. Top with the mashed avocado and tomato slices.

7. Serve.

Cooking Time: 10 minutes

Anti-Parkinson's Diet Dinner Recipes

1. Tofu Stir Fry

This vegan stir fry is packed with healthy ingredients and loaded with flavor. It's a great way to get a full serving of vegetables and protein in one dish.

Ingredients:

- 1 block of firm tofu, cut into cubes

- 2 tablespoons of olive oil

- 1 onion, diced

- 1 stripe-cut red bell pepper

- 2 minced garlic cloves

- 1 teaspoon of minced fresh ginger

- 2 teaspoons of soy sauce with reduced sodium

- 2 cups of broccoli florets

- 2 tablespoons of sesame oil

Instructions:

1. Set a sizable skillet over medium heat to preheat.

2. Add the olive oil and allow it to warm.

3. Add the tofu cubes to the skillet and cook for 8 minutes, stirring occasionally.

4. Add the onion, bell pepper, garlic, and ginger to the pan and cook for an additional 5 minutes.

5. Add the soy sauce and broccoli florets to the pan and cook for an additional 5 minutes.

6. Drizzle with sesame oil and serve.

Cooking Time: 18 minutes

2. Chickpea Curry

This cozy vegan curry is perfect for chilly nights. It is packed with nutritional benefits and the delicious flavor of curry.

Ingredients:

- 2 tablespoons of olive oil

- 1 onion, diced

- 2 cloves of garlic, minced

- 1 tablespoon of fresh ginger, minced

- 2 tablespoons of curry powder

- 1 can of rinsed and drained chickpeas

- 1 can of diced tomatoes

- 1 can of coconut milk

- 1 teaspoon of sea salt

- 1 tablespoon of lemon juice that has just been squeezed

- 1/4 cup of cilantro, chopped

Instructions:

1. Set a large pot over medium heat to preheat.

2. Add the olive oil and allow it to warm.

3. Add the onion, garlic, and ginger and cook for 5 minutes.

4. Add the curry powder and cook for an additional 2 minutes.

5. Add the chickpeas, diced tomatoes, coconut milk, sea salt, and lemon juice and bring to a simmer.

6. Simmer for 10 minutes.

7. Stir in the cilantro and serve.

Cooking Time: 17 minutes

3. Lentil Soup

This hearty vegan soup is packed with nutrition and flavor. It is the perfect meal for a cold night.

Ingredients:

- 2 tablespoons of olive oil

- 1 onion, diced

- 2 cloves of garlic, minced

- 1 teaspoon of fresh ginger, minced

- 2 cups of dry green lentils

- 4 cups of vegetable broth

- 1 teaspoon of sea salt

- 1/2 teaspoon of black pepper

Instructions:

1. Preheat a large pot over medium heat.

2. Add the olive oil and allow it to warm.

3. Add the onion, garlic, and ginger and cook for 5 minutes.

4. Add the lentils and vegetable broth and bring to a simmer.

5. Simmer for 25 minutes.

6. Add the sea salt and black pepper and stir to combine.

7. Serve.

Cooking Time: 30 minutes

4. Quinoa Bowl

This vegan bowl is packed with nutrition and flavor. It's a great way to get a full serving of vegetables and protein in one dish.

Ingredients:

- 1 cup of quinoa, cooked

- 2 tablespoons of olive oil

- 1 onion, diced

- 2 cloves of garlic, minced

- 1 teaspoon of fresh ginger, minced

- 1 red bell pepper, cut into strips

- 1 stripe-cut red bell pepper

- 1 cup of corn, frozen

- 2 teaspoons of soy sauce with reduced sodium

Instructions:

1. Preheat a large skillet over medium heat.

2. Add the olive oil and allow it to warm.

3. Add the onion, garlic, and ginger and cook for 5 minutes.

4. Add the bell pepper and corn and cook for an additional 5 minutes.

5. Add the cooked quinoa and soy sauce and stir to combine.

6. Heat for an additional 5 minutes.

7. Stir in the cilantro and serve.

Cooking Time: 15 minutes

5. Vegetable Fried Rice

This vegan fried rice is packed with vegetables and flavor. It is perfect for a quick, easy, and healthy dinner.

Ingredients:

- 2 tablespoons of olive oil

- 1 onion, diced

- 2 cloves of garlic, minced

- 1 teaspoon of fresh ginger, minced

- 2 cups of cooked brown rice

- 1 cup of frozen peas and carrots

- 2 teaspoons of soy sauce with reduced sodium

- 2 tablespoons of sesame oil

Instructions:

1. Set a sizable skillet over medium heat to preheat.

2. Stir in the olive oil, letting it warm.

3. Stir in the ginger, onion, and garlic, and simmer for 5 minutes.

4. Cook for a further 5 minutes after adding the cooked rice, frozen peas, and carrots.

5. Combine the soy sauce and sesame oil after adding them.

6. Heat for an additional 5 minutes.

7. Serve.

Cooking Time: 15 minutes

6. Baked Sweet Potatoes

This vegan baked sweet potatoes are packed with flavor and nutrition. They make a great side dish or light meal.

Ingredients:

- 4 sweet potatoes, washed and diced

- 2 tablespoons of olive oil

- 1 teaspoon of sea salt

- 1/2 teaspoon of black pepper

- 1 teaspoon of ground cumin

Instructions:

1. Preheat the oven to 400°F.

2. Set the sweet potatoes in dice on a baking sheet.

3. Drizzle with the olive oil and season with the sea salt, black pepper, and cumin.

4. Toss to coat.

5. Bake for 25 minutes.

6. Serve.

Cooking Time: 25 minutes

7. Vegetable Stir Fry

This vegan stir fry is packed with flavor and nutrition. It's a great way to get a full serving of vegetables in one dish.

Ingredients:

- 2 tablespoons of olive oil

- 1 onion, diced

- 2 cloves of garlic, minced

- 1 teaspoon of fresh ginger, minced

- 1 red bell pepper, cut into strips

- 1 stripe-cut red bell pepper

- 1 cup of frozen carrots and peas

- 2 teaspoons of soy sauce with reduced sodium

Instructions:

1. Set a sizable skillet over medium heat to preheat.

2. Add the olive oil and allow it to warm.

3. Add the onion, garlic, and ginger and cook for 5 minutes.

4. Add the bell pepper and peas and carrots and cook for an additional 5 minutes.

5. Combine the soy sauce and sesame oil after adding them.

6. Heat for an additional 5 minutes.

7. Serve.

Cooking Time: 15 minutes

8. Vegetable Curry

This vegan curry is a great way to get a full serving of vegetables in one dish. Both flavor and nutrition are abundant.

Ingredients:

- 2 tablespoons of olive oil

- 1 onion, diced

- 2 cloves of garlic, minced

- 1 tablespoon of fresh ginger, minced

- 2 tablespoons of curry powder

- 1 can of diced tomatoes

- 1 can of coconut milk

- 1 cup of frozen carrots and peas

- 1 tablespoon of freshly squeezed lemon juice

- 1 teaspoon of sea salt

- 1/4 cup of cilantro, chopped

Instructions:

1. Set a sizable pot over medium heat to preheat.

2. Add the olive oil and allow it to warm.

3. Add the onion, garlic, and ginger and cook for 5 minutes.

4. Add the curry powder and cook for an additional 2 minutes.

5. Add the diced tomatoes, coconut milk, peas and carrots, sea salt, and lemon juice and bring to a simmer.

6. Simmer for 10 minutes.

7. Stir in the cilantro and serve.

Cooking Time: 17 minutes

9. Roasted Vegetables

This vegan side dish is full of flavor and nutrition. Any meal would benefit from having it as a side dish.

Ingredients:

- 2 tablespoons of olive oil

- 1 onion, diced

- 2 cloves of garlic, minced

- 1 teaspoon of fresh ginger, minced

- 2 cups of diced vegetables (such as carrots, broccoli, and bell peppers)

- 1 teaspoon of sea salt

- 1/2 teaspoon of black pepper

Instructions:

1. Preheat the oven to 400°F.

2. Place the diced vegetables on a baking sheet.

3. Drizzle with the olive oil and season with the sea salt and black pepper.

4. Toss to coat.

5. Bake for 25 minutes.

6. Serve.

Cooking Time: 25 minutes

10. Vegetable Soup

This vegan soup is full of flavor and nutrition. It is the perfect meal for a night cold.

Ingredients:

- 2 tablespoons of olive oil

- 1 onion, diced

- 2 cloves of garlic, minced

- 1 teaspoon of fresh ginger, minced

- 4 cups of vegetable broth

- 1 can of diced tomatoes

- 1 cup of diced vegetables (such as carrots, broccoli, and bell peppers)

- 1 teaspoon of sea salt

- 1/2 teaspoon of black pepper

Instructions:

1. Set a sizable pot over medium heat to preheat.

2. Add the olive oil and allow it to warm.

3. Add the onion, garlic, and ginger and cook for 5 minutes.

4. Add the vegetable broth, diced tomatoes, diced vegetables, sea salt, and black pepper and bring to a simmer.

5. Simmer for 25 minutes.

6. Serve.

Cooking Time: 30 minutes

Anti-Parkinson's Diet Dessert Recipes

1. Apple Pie with Cinnamon Nutmeg Crumble Topping

Apple Pie with Cinnamon Nutmeg Crumble Topping is a delicious and healthy dessert for Parkinson's patients. This recipe is packed with antioxidants and anti-inflammatory properties to help reduce symptoms.

Ingredients:

- 4 apples, peeled and sliced

- 2 tablespoons of sugar

- 1 teaspoon of cinnamon

- 1 teaspoon of nutmeg

- 1/2 cup of all-purpose flour

- 1/2 cup of butter, melted

- 1/2 cup of chopped pecans

Instructions:

1. Preheat oven to 350°F.

2. In a large bowl, combine the apples, sugar, cinnamon, and nutmeg.

3. Place the mixture into an 8-inch pie pan.

4. In a medium bowl, mix together the flour, butter, and pecans until crumbly.

5. Sprinkle the crumble mixture over the apple mixture.

6. Bake for 40 to 45 minutes, or until golden brown on top.

Cooking Time: 40-45 minutes.

2. Mango Crisp

Mango Crisp is a simple and delicious dessert packed with vitamins and minerals to help manage symptoms of Parkinson's disease.

Ingredients:

- 4 ripe mangoes, peeled and chopped

- 1/2 cup of all-purpose flour

- 1/2 cup of oats

- 1/4 cup of brown sugar

- 1/4 cup of butter, melted

- 1 teaspoon of cinnamon

- 1/2 teaspoon of nutmeg

Instructions:

1. Preheat oven to 350°F.

2. Place the mangoes into an 8-inch baking dish.

3. In a medium bowl, mix together the flour, oats, brown sugar, butter, cinnamon, and nutmeg.

4. Sprinkle the mixture over the mangoes.

5. Bake for 40 to 45 minutes, or until golden brown on top.

Cooking Time: 40-45 minutes.

3. Blueberry Oat Bars

Blueberry Oat Bars are a delicious and healthy dessert that can help reduce the symptoms of Parkinson's disease.

This recipe is filled with antioxidants and anti-inflammatory properties.

Ingredients:

- 2 cups of rolled oats

- 1/2 cup of all-purpose flour

- 1/2 cup of brown sugar

- 1/2 teaspoon of baking powder

- 1/2 teaspoon of salt

- 1/2 cup of butter, melted

- 1 cup of fresh blueberries

Instructions:

1. Preheat oven to 350°F.

2. In a large bowl, mix together the oats, flour, brown sugar, baking powder, and salt.

3. Include the melted butter and stir to a crumbly consistency.

4. Press half of the mixture into an 8-inch baking dish.

5. Spread the blueberries over the crust.

6. Sprinkle the remaining oat mixture over the blueberries.

7. Bake for 40 to 45 minutes, or until golden brown on top.

Cooking Time: 40-45 minutes.

4. Carrot Cake with Cream Cheese Frosting

Carrot Cake with Cream Cheese Frosting is a delicious and healthy dessert for Parkinson's patients. This recipe is filled with vitamins and minerals to help reduce symptoms.

Ingredients:

- 2 cups of all-purpose flour

- 1 teaspoon of baking soda

- 1 teaspoon of baking powder

- 1 teaspoon of cinnamon

- 1/2 teaspoon of nutmeg

- 1/2 teaspoon of salt

- 1/2 cup of butter, melted

- 1/2 cup of brown sugar

- 2 eggs

- 2 cups of grated carrots

- 1/2 cup of chopped walnuts

- 8 ounces of cream cheese, softened

- 1/2 cup of powdered sugar

Instructions:

1. Preheat oven to 350°F.

2. In a large bowl, mix together the flour, baking soda, baking powder, cinnamon, nutmeg, and salt.

3. In a separate bowl, mix together the butter, brown sugar, eggs, and carrots.

4. Combine the dry ingredients with the liquid components after adding them.

5. Stir in the walnuts.

6. Spread the mixture into an 8-inch baking dish.

7. Bake for 40-45 minutes, or until a toothpick inserted into the center comes out clean.

8. In a medium bowl, mix together the cream cheese and powdered sugar.

9. Spread the cream cheese frosting over the cake.

Cooking Time: 40-45 minutes.

5. Banana Bread

Banana Bread is a healthy and delicious dessert for Parkinson's patients. This recipe is filled with fiber and vitamins to help reduce symptoms.

Ingredients:

- 2 cups of all-purpose flour

- 1 teaspoon of baking soda

- 1/2 teaspoon of salt

- 1/2 cup of butter, melted

- 1/2 cup of brown sugar

- 2 eggs

- 3 ripe bananas, mashed

- 1/2 cup of chopped walnuts

Instructions:

1. Preheat oven to 350°F.

2. Combine the flour, baking soda, and salt in a big bowl.

3. Combine the butter, brown sugar, eggs, and mashed bananas in another bowl.

4. Combine the dry ingredients with the liquid components after adding them.

5. Stir in the walnuts.

6. Spread the mixture into an 8-inch baking dish.

7. Bake for 40-45 minutes, or until a toothpick inserted into the center comes out clean.

Cooking Time: 40-45 minutes.

Anti-Parkinson's Diet Snack Recipes

1. Banana and Oat Muffins

This recipe is a great way to eat healthy snacks while helping to fight Parkinson's. It includes bananas, oats, and other healthy ingredients.

Ingredients:

- 1/2 cup sugar

- 1/2 cup vegetable oil

- 2 eggs

- 1 cup mashed banana

- 1 1/2 cups all-purpose flour

- 1 teaspoon baking soda

- 1 teaspoon baking powder

- 1/2 teaspoon salt

- 1 cup oats

Instructions:

1. Preheat your oven to 375°F.

2. In a large bowl, whisk together the sugar, oil, and eggs.

3. Add the mashed banana and mix until combined.

4. In a separate bowl, mix together the flour, baking soda, baking powder, and salt.

5. Add the dry ingredients to the wet ingredients and mix until just combined.

6. Fold in the oats.

7. Grease a muffin tin with non-stick spray and fill each cavity with the batter.

8. Bake for 15-20 minutes, or until a toothpick inserted into the center of a muffin comes out clean.

Cooking Time: 15-20 minutes

2. Sweet Potato Fries

These sweet potato fries are an easy and delicious way to get a nutrient-packed snack while helping to fight Parkinson's.

Ingredients:

- 2 large sweet potatoes, cut into French fry-sized pieces

- 1 tablespoon olive oil

- 1/2 teaspoon garlic powder

- 1/2 teaspoon paprika

- 1/4 teaspoon salt

- 1/4 teaspoon pepper

Instructions:

1. Preheat your oven to 425°F.

2. Place the sweet potato pieces in a bowl and drizzle with the olive oil.

3. Sprinkle the garlic powder, paprika, salt, and pepper over the sweet potatoes and stir until evenly coated.

4. Place the sweet potatoes on a baking sheet lined with parchment paper.

5. Bake for 20 minutes, or until the potatoes are golden brown and crispy.

Cooking Time: 20 minutes

3. Roasted Chickpeas

These roasted chickpeas are a great source of protein while also helping to fight Parkinson's.

Ingredients:

- 2 cans chickpeas, drained and rinsed

- 2 tablespoons olive oil

- 1 teaspoon garlic powder

- 1 teaspoon paprika

- 1/2 teaspoon salt

- 1/2 teaspoon pepper

Instructions:

1. Preheat your oven to 400°F.

2. Place the chickpeas in a bowl and drizzle with the olive oil.

3. Sprinkle the garlic powder, paprika, salt, and pepper over the chickpeas and stir until evenly coated.

4. Place the chickpeas on a baking sheet lined with parchment paper.

5. Bake for 15-20 minutes, or until the chickpeas are golden brown and crispy.

Cooking Time: 15-20 minutes

4. Fruit Salad

This fruit salad is packed with vitamins and antioxidants that can help to fight Parkinson's.

Ingredients:

- 1/2 cup blueberries

- 1/2 cup strawberries, sliced

- 1/2 cup blackberries

- 1/2 cup raspberries

- 1/2 cup diced mango

- 2 tablespoons honey

Instructions:

1. In a large bowl, mix together the blueberries, strawberries, blackberries, raspberries, and mango.

2. Drizzle the honey over the fruit and stir until evenly coated.

3. Serve immediately, or store in the refrigerator for up to 3 days.

Cooking Time: 0 minutes

5. Avocado Toast

This simple and delicious avocado toast is a great way to get healthy fats while helping to fight Parkinson's.

Ingredients:

- 2 slices of whole wheat bread

- 1 ripe avocado, mashed

- 1/4 teaspoon garlic powder

- 1/4 teaspoon paprika

- 1/4 teaspoon salt

Instructions:

1. Toast the bread in a toaster or in a skillet over medium heat.

2. In a small bowl, mash the avocado and mix in the garlic powder, paprika, and salt.

3. Spread the mashed avocado over the toast and serve.

Cooking Time: 5 minutes

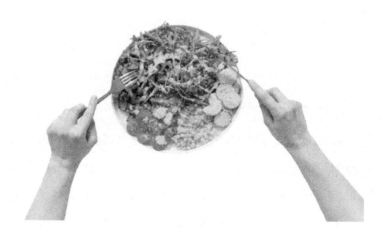

Conclusion

In conclusion, an anti-Parkinson's diet is an important part of helping to manage the symptoms of Parkinson's disease. Eating a balanced diet that is high in fiber, low in fat, and moderate in protein can help reduce the severity of Parkinson's symptoms while also promoting overall health. Additionally, avoiding caffeine, alcohol, processed foods, and certain medications can also be beneficial.

While there is no one-size-fits-all diet for everyone with Parkinson's, following these dietary guidelines can help reduce symptoms and improve quality of life. With the right diet, it is possible to enjoy a healthier and more fulfilling life despite having Parkinson's disease.

In addition to dietary modifications, it is also important to exercise regularly and to remain socially engaged. Exercise can help increase mobility and reduce muscle stiffness, while socialization can help reduce feelings of isolation and depression.

By combining dietary changes, exercise, and socialization, those living with Parkinson's can improve their quality of life and have a better overall experience.

Overall, an anti-Parkinson's diet is an important part of managing the disease. With a few dietary modifications and lifestyle changes, it is possible to reduce the severity of symptoms and live a more fulfilling life.

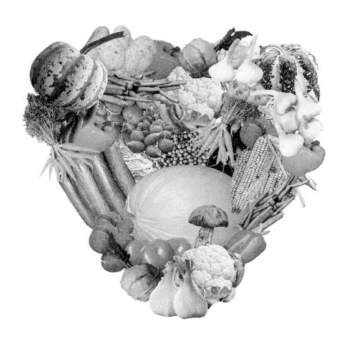

Printed in Great Britain
by Amazon

36884386R00066